FASCINATION AURA SURGERY

Angelika Schlinger

Copyright © 2014 Angelika Schlinger

December 2014

All rights reserved

Translation by Stefanie Colbert

faszinationaurachirurgie@gmail.com

ISBN: 1505549434
ISBN-13: 978-1505549430

PRELIMINARY MARK OF THE AUTHOR

I have reviewed the here presented information and particularly the method of aura surgery to the best of our knowledge and belief. The practice of aura surgery is not suitable for people who have had no training in the correct use of this method. Therefore, I assume no liability for damages of any kind that result directly or indirectly from the utilization of this information or the method of aura surgery by Gerhard Klügl. Any liability of the author for damage to health or to people is precluded. In the case of doubt, especially with physical or mental illnesses, I recommend visiting a doctor or naturopath. The here represented method does not replace treatments by a medical practitioner or naturopath, nor the medicines prescribed by a medical practitioner or naturopath.

Original Edition October 2014

Contents

FOREWORD BY GERHARD KLÜGL..........................viii

PROLOG 1

MY PATH TO THE AURA SURGERY............................3

THE JOURNEY BEGINS..5

FIRST EXPERIENCES WITH THE QUANTUM FIELD..7

LET MIRACLES HAPPEN: QUANTUM PHYSICS FOR EVERYONE..9

CASE 1: AURA SURGERY ON A FEMALE ROTTWEILER..13

QUANTUM ENTANGLEMENT: SYMPTOMS FROM ETERNITY 16

CHRISTINE, 22 – OBSESSINAL WASHING, ANXIETIES AND ECZEMA ON BOTH HANDS 18

PETER, 46 – A TEAR IN THE LUNG OUT OF NOWHERE 20

NOT ALWAYS MYSTICAL: INJURIES IN THE PRESENT LIFE..22

GISELA, NO AGE – CATARACT..................................25

MELANIE, EARLY 20'S – TEAR IN THE CORNEA .28

PLACEBO-EFFECT – YOUR METABOLISM BELIEVES IN YOU 30

RENATE, EARLY 60'S – CHRONIC STOMACH PAINS SINCE CHILDHOOD 35

MATTER – ENERGY – INFORMATION – EMOTION 37

ROLAND, 58 – ROOFER (AGAIN) WITH FARSIGHTEDNESS 40

GABI, 50 - DIAPHRAGMATIC HERNIA 42

NOCEBO – THE IMAGINARY INVALID 45

KERSTIN, 42 – BENDY LEG CORRECTION „WITHOUT THE LOWER LEG" 48

KERSTIN SUBSEQUENT TREATMENT – FINALLY TAKING A PART IN LIFE 51

WHEN DIAGNONES KILL 54

INVESTIGATED – A HEART ATTACK IS NO CANCER 57

DISTANT HEALING – QUANTUM ENTANGLEMENT IN ACTION 60

DR. JUR. ERNST PECHTL – DISTANT HEALING LUMBAR SPINE 62

KATRIN, 50 – TENNIS INSTEAD OF ARM SLING .64

HOW MANY TIMES? – ALWAYS REBIRTH 67

KARIN, 45 – DIED FOR THE SCOTTISH CLAN: ONLY WHO KNOWS THE RULES CAN REALLY PLAY 69

MARY, MID 50'S – I FEEL CHANGED 72

„THE ARGUMENT, LIVING ORGANISMS ARE ONLY ELPAINABLE THROUGH THE LAWS OF PHYSICS AND THE VITALITY OF POWER DOES NOT EXIST, DOES NOT CORRESPOND WITH THE MODERN QUANTUM THEORY." 74

LAW OF THE RESONANCE OR – MONEY MAKES MONEY 76

GERDA, 49 – SINGLE MOM RIPE FOR A VACATION 78

THE CIRCLE CLOSES – OFF TO NEW WATERS 80

CONTACT AND EXCHANGE OF IDEAS 82

THANK YOU 83

BIBLIOGRAPHY 84

ABOUT THE AUTHOR 85

For Dad, because he already got me into contact with „the energy" when I was learning how to read and write. Thank you very much. Now I know what you meant by this!

FOREWORD BY GERHARD KLÜGL

Aura surgery! If one comes across this term for the first time, one will think about faith healing, esoterism. Indeed, the aura as a term is used in the esoteric, but the aura is the subtle energy field that surrounds every object and every living thing.

When I had started using the aura surgery in 1998, it was already very difficult for me to classify this in my usual familiar technical thinking (Note from the author: Gerhard Klügl was as an official in the German Patent Office and later worked as a self-employed expert in the field of patent search. Today, in his second professional life, he works as an aura surgeon, astrologer, building biologist, medium and international healer from Liechtenstein. Since 2003 he is a member of the Biophysical Medicine Association (GBM) and winner of the European Medicine Prize of the Dr. Ingebort Gebert-Heiß-Foundation 2005).

When doctors began to be interested in this, I knew that aura surgery, for which I use surgical instruments and anatomical pictures or models, is better located in the field of science rather than esoteric.

Experiments in 2001 with Prof. Gary Schwartz at the university in Tucson/Arizona have proven that every step during the treatment with aura surgery was traceable with Kirlian photography. Also, measurements with high-precision scales that were performed from 2012 with the scientist Dr. Klaus Volkamer, clearly showed physical results. In treated individuals, weight changes, sometimes up to several kilograms were detected.

While implementing aura surgery, the search for the cause always stands in the first place. It is precisely the same approach that too applies to the classical homeopathy. The symptom is the path to the cause.

Over five years ago I have started to share this method of aura surgery with doctors and naturopaths. This is also how I got to know and appreciate Angelika Schlinger, as she completed and successfully passed the aura surgery training with me.

I am pleased that Angelika, as a classical homeopath, has so successfully integrated the aura surgery into her everyday practice. My goal is to be able to represent this new method to as many people as possible. Therefore, I thank Angelika for the examples of the successful use of aura surgery featured in her book. I wish Angelika Schlinger much success and that the book reaches many interested readers.

Gerhard F. Klügl
Ruggell, August 21st 2014

scientist Dr. Klaus Volkamer, clearly showed physical results. In treated individuals, weight changes, sometimes up to several kilograms were detected.

While implementing aura surgery, the search for the cause always stands in the first place. It is precisely the same approach that too applies to the classical homeopathy. The symptom is the path to the cause.

Over five years ago I have started to share this method of aura surgery with doctors and naturopaths. This is also how I got to know and appreciate Angelika Schlinger, as she completed and successfully passed the aura surgery training with me.

I am pleased that Angelika, as a classical homeopath, has so successfully integrated the aura surgery into her everyday practice. My goal is to be able to represent this new method to as many people as possible. Therefore, I thank Angelika for the examples of the successful use of aura surgery featured in her book. I wish Angelika Schlinger much success and that the book reaches many interested readers.

Gerhard F. Klügl
Ruggell, August 21st 2014

PROLOG

This book tells my experiences with the aura surgery after Gerhard Klügl. You do not know what that is? Aura surgery is a healing method, which doesn't treat the patient's physical body, but their subtle body, their aura. It is a surgical operation in the aura.

Because everything is connected to everything according to the quantum physics, impressive results can often be achieved with aura surgery. So impressive that not only Gisela, a particular patient of mine, urges for more people to get to know aura surgery. So, I tell you about Gisela now. Moreover, some other people like her, who like to tell their story to introduce this healing method to other persons.

I am practising as a naturopath in Germany. However, in Germany it may have legal consequences when a healer publicly describes "successful" treatments or even speaks of cured patients.

Therefore, I would like to point out:

1. I do not claim that the aura surgery heals people. For this, I am waiting for significant scientific evidence (as you know from Gerhard of Klügl's foreword, (not just) he is working on it). However, if a patient claims that he experienced relieve or even cure through aura surgery, I

will not call him a liar. Moreover, in this book I gladly make some pages available for the personal and subjective experience reports of some of my patients.

2. I explicitly state that the described cases are individual cases and not transferable to others or even more general that the relief of the described symptoms is to be generalized - because every person is unique. In every way. Therefore, healers, doctors or naturopaths are not generally allowed to make a promise of healing, even if he has already successfully treated something similar in practice.

3. I agree with the critics and skeptics out there that think that many or possibly all "successful" cases of aura surgery relate to placebo effects. Placebo effects occur when an individual heals "itself" because it has great emotional confidence in its therapist, the form of treatment and the own self-healing powers. In the book, more thoughts on the topic can be found in the chapter "Placebo effect: your metabolism believes in you". Personally, I am a big fan of placebo effects. Hereby I encourage to officially place placebo effects into the ailing health care system as side-effect free, cost-effective and commonly available "medication".

By the way, I believe that there is no doctor, healer, shaman or any other healer that can restore the health of people. We all can only point our patients into the direction of how to gain access to the self-healing powers again.

Nobody except god alone can restore another person's health. Everyone is allowed to become healthy on their own.here.

MY PATH TO THE AURA SURGERY

"There is no way you will be able to get a seat in this seminar. I am totally booked out, and the waiting list is full until at least Easter." The resolute woman on the phone was Andrea D. with whom I really wanted to complete an advanced training in the medial field.

Mediality, to be a medium. It sounds so esoteric or as my son would say „spacey".

I am a naturopath and actually really down to earth. In my practice of alternative medicine, I have worked many years in classical homeopathy and the pure material orthomolecular therapy, which is the use of vitamins and minerals. I am very satisfied with the combination of the construction plan and building material to develop a healthy organism. My patients are so enthusiastic that I don't have to search for new patients because through word of mouth they come to me on their own.

Then I have discovered quantum physics. For me, as a naturopath, quantum physics also mean quantum medicine. For 20 years I have had a pleasant experience with classical homeopathy, the healing out of "nowhere", respectively out of a few sugar pallets. Quantum medicine is even less, like homeopathy without globules. The healing out of "nowhere" – is that the progression?

I wanted to know. Moreover, it should not be Mrs. D.,

my selected favorite. So, I was frustrated when I went online to search for an alternative. The offerings were nearly endless, but nothing was at least a little matching for me.

I was enervated and wanted to take a break with music video on YouTube.

Instead, a window popped up with a short video about some Mr. Klügl, who treated a client in his aura. He was chopping and fumbling about 20 centimeters away from his "patient's" body, who in turn eagerly gave feedback. "It still aches here, oh, it stings… Yes, now it is better." It almost looked ridiculous to me; should I really take this serious?

Mr. Klügl himself seemed anything, but ridiculous; an older man with high seriousness and the balance of a person that is absolutely sure about what he is doing. So I kept googling about this charismatic man, and I landed on a web page, where a Klügl-seminar on the subject mediality was offered from Mrs. Kellermann in Munich. I called.

"Actually, the seminar has been fully booked for weeks", said Brigitte Kellermann. „But someone has canceled just 2 minutes ago. If that works, then that is how it should be; if you like you can have the spot." Of course, I wanted it.

So I drove to the seminar „Mediality" with Gerhard Klügl, the father of aura surgery. Apart from my stressful everyday practice life and all the nice conversation with the other interesting participants, I looked forward to a relaxing weekend.

It turned out quite differently.

THE JOURNEY BEGINS

I already arrived 3 hours prior to the beginning of the seminar. After I brought my luggage into the room, I suddenly felt crushed. I wanted to lay on the bed for a little while, and then go to the seminar room early so I could meet Mr. Klügl and a few of the participants before the beginning of the seminar.

Instead, I fell into a narcotic sleep. When I woke up, my watch read 5:10 pm. The seminar started 10 minutes ago. I rushed into the seminar room, almost all seats in the circle were taken by observant listeners. Mr. Klügl did not interrupt his opening word, quickly nodded at me and then asked the other participants to introduce themselves to the group. This way the embarrassment of my disturbance was kept within limits. But it wasn't about to get better.

Shortly before it was my turn to introduce myself, I again felt unbelievably crushed. In addition, I suddenly felt a pressure on my chest as if it came from a boulder. I could barely breathe and at the same time I felt panic rising in me, which forced me to take flight out of the seminar room.

I stopped and stood in front of the door as if I was in a trance. After, what seemed like an eternity, I noticed a supporting hand and calming words coming from a woman. She introduced herself as Brigitte Kellermann.

The friendly seminar organizer from Munich. „That was impetuous", she said calmly and smiled. „Come with me into my room, it's right over there."

After a glass of water and a treatment, that looked similar to what I already knew from the online video with Gerhard Klügl, I felt much better.

I apologized to my helper and told her that this is not usually the way I get myself noticed. Brigitte explained to me that it „just sometimes happens that specific energies do not like it when someone develops energetically." „It is usually a positive sign; you probably have a talent to do good", She said lapidary. And the panic started to rise in me again.

The next thing I remembered is Gerhard Klügl's face. In the air, he moved his hands around my neck and chest, and calmly talked to me. I felt better by the minute, the panic reduced and I felt comfortable and if I was in good hands.

Mr. Klügl shared Brigitte's view. „This was something energetic!" he said determined. „It can happen if someone is indeed open to things like these. Just good you first came to the mediality-seminar. I wouldn't have that much time during aura surgery training." He coolly turned to the door. „I have to go to the seminar. We will see each other later." And I felt fantastic.

This is how my personal experience with the aura surgery came faster than expected. Instead of having to wait for months for an appointment with Gerhard Klügl, he came to me. Spontaneous and without notice. And, I was able to directly experience the unbelievable effectiveness of the aura surgery.

Now if this wasn't a good omen…

FIRST EXPERIENCES WITH THE QUANTUM FIELD

However, I was able to enjoy the longer part of the mediality seminar. I learned how to protect myself against energetic attackers and how I set myself in the oscillations of objects and to even recognize snapshots from the lives of their earlier and current owners.

A few practical exercises helped us with that, so one of Mr. Klügl's assistants handed me a spoon and asked me to feel it. "Just see if something happens, like pictures, feelings or anything."

After I held the spoon in my hands for a while, I „saw" the image of a middle-aged woman in front of me. She wore a dress in 1900s style and seemed to be a confident and independent woman.
This woman apparently lived in a town with a view of massive mountains. It was summer and she appeared to write a book about traveling to foreign and exotic countries.

The image got blurry and a different one appeared. This time it was a young woman that was dressed like a bride. She too seemed like a confident personality and one thing was clear: she did not want to marry the groom.

Before I was able to delve deeper into this feeling,

Gerhard Klügl stopped the exercise and asked us for our experiences. I told about the images that I have seen and I was surprised by the similarity to the real story of the spoon, that Karina, the assistant told us after:

The spoon belonged to her great-great-grandmother. She lived in Austria around the turn of the 20th century. She operated a retail store in the capital city of Vienna. She dreamed of traveling to foreign countries like India but because the financial situation did not allow it she wrote novels that took place there.

Karina received the spoon from her grandmother as a wedding gift. However, the marriage never took place. She chose not to marry her fiance a couple of days before the ceremony.

So, is it really possible to get information about another time era from a physical spoon? Esoteric nonsense or basic knowledge of quantum physics? Let's ask an expert:

„For us believing in physicists", wrote Albert Einstein "the distinction between past, present and future is only a stubbornly persistent illusion."

I was bound to develop into a „believing physicist". I was fascinated with my experiences and a just a short time after, I enrolled in aura surgery training.

Oh yes, of course, the seminar was booked out. But I ignored that fact and therefore still became a spot. I will explain to you shortly how that works.

LET MIRACLES HAPPEN: QUANTUM PHYSICS FOR EVERYONE

The quantum physics as well as the aura surgery assume that all known knowledge is already available, stored in the so-called quantum field. This information is not reserved to an elite group of spiritual gurus, but available for everyone. As long as he admits to this quantum field and focusses his entire concentration on a certain point.

"What are Quanta?" you ask justifiably. Well, quanta are actually the smallest portions of the reality that surrounds us. The portions that are no longer divisible; at least not in the current state of our science. I deliberately call them portions and not particles, because a quantum is sometimes a particle and sometimes a wave. This realization, that every matter (electrons, protons, atoms, molecules,...) does not only possess particle property, but can also be described as a wave is one of the most important achievements of modern physics. Thereof it deduces a central sentence of quantum physics, that is: "The energy follows the attention."

Werner Karl Heisenberg, one of the most important physicists of the twentieth century, postulated this theory in its uncertainty relation. It means that the current location and the velocity of a particle can never be measured at the same time. It can only be decided by measuring it, whether it is a particle in a limited space (place) or a wave, which extends over wide spaces (speed).

Or to say it with an example (borrowed from the cellular biologist Bruce Lipton): these quanta are like your teen sons and daughters; either you know, where they (statically) reside (e.g. on the sofa in front of the TV) or they move themselves (in a discotheque, a club or such, where you're not with them). You will fail to observe them at the same time at a specific place and during a specific, measurable movement of your choice (e.g. mowing the lawn in the parental garden).

But the phenomenon does not exist out of itself, but only in correlation with an observer and the observer's expectations. Which in this case it's you.
A different observer with other experiences and other expectations would certainly produce a different result. Difficult to understand? Well, actually it's quite simple.

Well, you probably assume already from the outset that you can't get your son off the sofa anyway. Your experiences from the past few months steer your expectations. The interaction with another observer, for example a friend of your son, will certainly bring other results...

Which in turn means the observer: "By observing something, as in focusing, I am creating it." In plain terms: whatever you concentrate on (by expecting it) will occur. Simpler worded: You create your own reality. (It only works to a limited extent with the teenagers example; as always, exceptions prove the rule).

Try it out: There is never free parking in front of your favorite local pub? And you know that, because you have to park 2 blocks further every time. You already think about it when starting driving from home: "Oh man, it's absolutely bucketing down. I guarantee I won't find a parking spot nearby again. I am probably soaking wet when I finally arrive at the pub." And prompt, it happens (again)?

If you're going today, tell yourself instead: "Awesome. Exactly when I arrive, someone will leave. I will park directly in front of the pub and also my favorite table is still available inside. I'm a lucky kid!" Do this with real enjoyment and you will see promptly that that's what happens. Because you have focused on one of your favorite parking spots.

In the aura surgery we focus our attention on the aura, which is the subtle body of our patients. And if we get involved with these patients, to a certain extent we can make his aura statically detectable for our subtle touch.

In this process, it is imperative for the aura surgeon to approach a patient completely neutral. This is probably one of the hardest exercises for us humans. However, we strongly tend to assign and generalize a once made experience immediately onto similar cases.

During my training at Gerhard Klügl, I learned to focus and to feel the aura of my patients, which I could only see before.
When the patient goes into resonance with me, then a treatment in the aura is possible, in the subtle range. This treatment is not magic. It is "just" the exchange of information between two parties. The quantum physic has an explanation: the quantum entanglement.

Simpler worded: two particles meet at some point during their trip, exchange views and when they again proceed on different paths, they still remain in contact all the time. These particles thereby share their vigorous conditions and their information. And that happens in real-time (synchronicity is the technical term, if you ever wanted to brag with this). So right now.

By the way, this is also the simple and logical explanation of the functioning of distant healings. Exchange of information in the quantum field. Again a magic was physically revealed. How unromantic.

Back to the aura surgery. Before a treatment, I sense the aura of my patients, which I mostly feel about 20 cm away from his body. Thereby I completely focus on the vibration of the patients, to track down energetic blockages.

A blockage usually shows itself, when my hands really cling to his aura. A clear information, which I then need to decipher with the help of my patients.

A person also often has physical complaints there, where blockages show up in the aura. And then I can send the needed healing information to my patient through the entangled quantum. His cells then integrate this information and then the symptom, which the patient suffers from, can be fixed.

For those who want to know more: The book from the American biologist Bruce Lipton, with the theme "Intelligent Cells", explains the backgrounds. Based on scientific insights about the biochemical functions of our body, he shows that our personal life as well as our collective coexistence are controlled by the connection between mind and matter.

As far as the theory, that I understood and found to be logical. The fourth seminar block in my training to be an aura surgeon was standing right around the corner. I looked forward to it. But before being able to take part, I was taught to master my first practical challenge.

CASE 1: AURA SURGERY ON A FEMALE ROTTWEILER

We live together with a female dog. She is a Rottweiler-Shepherd mix, and listens (most of the time) to the name Meggi. During our seminars and trips, Meggi stays in a hotel for dogs in our proximity.

A few days before the start of the fourth aura surgery seminar, Meggi began to rip apart her pillow and started to build a nest. She was more affectionate than usual and no longer left my side. When I drove to my practice, she did not eat or drink until I was back home. She kept her ball, which she usually brings for us to throw and play with, and herded it like an infant. In short: Meggi was pseudo pregnant!

In this state, I couldn't bring her to the dog hotel; but I also could not take her to the seminar. And in contrast to usual, she showed no reaction to the carefully selected homeopathic remedies.

Great, I had created my first case. You remember the law: "The energy follows the attention"? Here it is in its purest form: I was thinking of my training to be an aura surgeon. I was pretty unsure whether I could actually do that right. And how should I start, what case would be simple enough that I could use as my first practice case... Obviously, this case was it.

FASCINATION AURA SURGERY

So, my first major surgery in the aura was now imminent. Diagnosis: pseudo pregnancy in a 9 year old Rottweiler, homeopathy resistant. Therapy: aura surgical scraping.

Well, it's one thing to do the training to be an aura surgeon at Gerhard Klügls together with other practitioners and doctors. But alone at home, it is a completely different thing to implement what you learned into action, without too much doubt on the method and my ability to implement them.

Despite my years of work in the field of energy medicine, I am not free of questioning the methods every now and again. To test their reliability. And from conversations with many therapists, I know that this phenomenon is common even among the most successful colleagues.

With a healthy respect I prepared my surgical instruments and brought Meggi to me. Because we maintain an honest dealing together, I told her about the upcoming operation and the hoped-for result. She laid next to me and dozed off.

I palpated Meggi's aura, the way I had learned it at Gerhards. I was not sure I could actually feel a blockage in her womb or had I imagined it? Whatever.

Either the aura surgery is complete nonsense and at worst nothing happens, or it is a functioning therapy. In this case, after many years of practical experience and training to be an aura surgeon, I have enough knowledge to perform the operation.

I imagined Meggi's anatomy plastically. Then I began the operation in the aura, well, "in the air", about 20 cm away from Meggi's physical body. First I shaved genitals and thighs in her aura, in some distance from her body, and disinfected them with an energetic iodine solution.

With visualized clamps I retained the external os of the uterus, then I carefully widened the cervix.
(At this point I'd like to thank YouTube, where I had found a film that has helped me a lot. Because until now, as a natural health professional for humans, I had little idea of the anatomy of a female dog.)

Then I gently scraped out the cervix and uterine cavity with a sharp instrument and removed the endometrium. Everything happened in her aura of course; I haven't touched her physical body!

Meggi had not moved throughout the entire operation. She laid next to me completely quiet and relaxed and it even seemed that she enjoyed the surgery.
I, on the other hand, was highly concentrated and tense. The well-being of my dog and the participation in the seminar were at stake. I can see you smile in disbelief. But wait, it gets better!

After the finishing act, we both slept for a little while. After an hour, I was awakened by Meggi. She had her ball in the mouth and pushed me. She wanted me to throw the ball and play with her. She also didn't built a nest anymore and when I came home in the evening after a few hours at the practice, she had completely emptied her food bowl.

My first aura surgery operation was a success!

The pseudo pregnancy was done with, Meggi was able to go the dog hotel and I was able to go to the Gerhard Klügl seminar. It could go on this way!

QUANTUM ENTANGLEMENT: SYMPTOMS FROM ETERNITY

We already know that Albert Einstein considered the linear time an illusion and also today's scientists share this opinion.

The german physicist Prof. Dr. Markolf Niemz hypothesizes in his book „Lucy with c" that the concept of eternity includes all time eras. That explicitly includes the time after the physical death. Inter alia, this is how he describes this:

"As seen from earth, time elapses for everything that does not travel with the speed of light. Consequently, also for the soul that spreads with the speed of light. So if our soul is actually accelerated to the speed of light after the physical death (Note: that is what he has hypothetically proven in the previous text), then time stands still for the soul – as seen from earth. The theology has characterized one term that precisely describes this state: Eternity".

The information on the life after death are saved to the memory of the soul and are, thanks to the quantum entanglement, passed on to the cells of the body in real time with the next materialization (reincarnation, which means: "becoming-meat-again"). And that is where these informations are integrated into the life. Negative and positive, from the point of view of a person that currently lives this life.

Is it possible for some people to have a particular intensive memory of specific abilities? Maybe it is this memorized knowledge, which was acquired in the past life that makes these people to child prodigies? In this way, it could be explained why Wolfgang Amadeus Mozart published his first compositions at only the age 5 and at the age of 6 first concert tours were organized for this child prodigy.

And this is the explanation, that also the cause is to be searched reversible for physical and/or psychological symptoms in a "murderous" incident from the past life, that adopted itself in the energetic memory?

For example, like it happened to Christine.

CHRISTINE, 22 – OBSESSINAL WASHING, ANXIETIES AND ECZEMA ON BOTH HANDS

Christine is a 22-year-old young woman. Over the past few years she has developed ablutomania, which mainly related to her hands. Not too long ago, the skin of her hands were dark red, completely dry and chapped past her wrists. This is how Christine describes the feeling: „They burn like fire. But I constantly have the feeling that they are somehow dirty, and boiling".

Christine is a vegetarian since the age of 9 because the smell particularly of roasted meat causes her severe nausea. She clearly dislikes the USA in spite of the fact that she has never been there. A trip to the United States is out of the question.

She has great respect for electricity: „It gives me the creeps when I have to change a light bulb."

In 1890, the first person was executed by the electric chair. To this day this form of legalized killing is practiced in the USA. For this, the death row inmates are strapped down with leather straps on their feet, chest and stomach and above the wrists.

In an interview in October 2010 with the german

newspaper "Frankfurter Rundschau", a former
executioner describes the smell of the execution „as if a fat
ham is roasted."

I let Christine symbolically sit down in the electric chair.
She immediately became very pale and began to breathe
shallowly but really fast. Symbolically I pulled the plug
from the electricity grid and in her aura I removed the
metal cap from her head as well as a contact from her right
lower leg; those are the two things that are responsible for
the electric shock through the entire body of the death row
inmate. I symbolically cut through the leather straps with
which her forearms were strapped down above her wrists.
Next, I let her get up and purposefully let her leave the cell
of her execution.

After the aura surgical removal of the trauma cause, it is of
particular importance to restore the affected body
functions of the patient. In Christine case is was primarily
her psychological condition, her obsessional washing and
her disgust for roasted meat. Secondly, a couple of inner
organs like her were affected.
It took a good hour until all functions were restored.

Christine called me the next day and told me the following:
„The obsessional washing slightly got better. I walked by a
food stall today and steaks were grilled there. The smell did
not bother me and the best of all: My hands are neither red
nor inflamed anymore!!!"
The results of the aura surgical intervention with Christine
were recognizable through the change of her health
condition. Sometimes during an aura surgery session we
find signs in retrospect that could explain an already
overcome illness or accident from the present life.

Like it happened with Peter.

PETER, 46 – A TEAR IN THE LUNG OUT OF NOWHERE

Peter is a 40-year-old contractor. With jeans, t-shirt, and his slightly gray shoulder-length hair he seems more like a freedom-loving biker that cruises through the country as a „lonely rider", then an economic oriented businessman.

Peter does not come to the practice because of specific complaints, but „just out of interest for the aura surgery". He acts open-minded and yet a bit derisive which can refer to both, my work and to me as a person.

It does not matter if someone takes the aura surgery serious or not. It also does not matter if the patient „believes in it" or not. The quantum field really does not care if a person believes in it or not. But according to my experiences it is an enormous advantage during aura surgical operations when a patient is able to feel something in any type of form while being treated in his aura. This is not really necessary to get a changed result, but the advantage for a positive outcome is probably undisputed among my aura surgery colleagues.

It is hard to assess Peter. Does he really mean what he says or are his reactions to my questions sarcastic?

I cannot seize him in his aura until I felt a blockage at the height of the chest in the right lung. It feels as if a piece of metal is stuck in his lung between the lower ribs.

Simultaneously I see the image of a young pilot in front of me, he is alone and is sitting in an out-dated fighter plane. He is in his mid-twenties and is wearing a leather cap. He is hit by shrapnel or something similar and a piece of metal is stuck in his lung. It is impossible for him to breathe and he died before the crashing airplane hits the ground.

I tell Peter about the images, aura surgically remove the metal splinter, attended his wound and closed it. When I was finished, Peter said that, in his present life, "my lung tore just because I moved something. The doctor said it was a spontaneous reaction of my body and it could have happened even while sleeping."

Peter lifted up his shirt and showed me the long scar, which is the result of the lung operation. This scar was exactly on the line where the shrapnel had penetrated the costal arch and the lungs of the young pilot.
Peter was 21 years old when his lung tore.

NOT ALWAYS MYSTICAL: INJURIES IN THE PRESENT LIFE

The aura surgery is not just an alternative healing method for injuries of the past life but is also is excellent for profane symptoms caused from the present time.

Why? Firstly, because –as we already know- the energy follows the attention. And secondly, because we do not only consist of matter. On the contrary.

But, of how much matter do we consist of? Let's do a rough calculation:

Our body consists of cells and these, in logical consequent, of atoms. The diameter of the various atoms ranges in the ballpark of 10^{-10} m, their mass ranges from 10^{-27} to 10^{-25} kg. The nanoscale is 10^{-9}, which is 1 billionth. And at 10^{-10} we have a range of 10 billionth.

A nucleus is 10.000 times smaller than the whole atom. The volume conforms to the third potency, so the space of the nucleus is one billion times less than the space that the entire atom claims (the volumes of the electrons are practically 0). Which means, a 10 billionth percent.

Can you picture these dimensions? Neither can I!

But, if you would pack all of the masses of your body

as tightly together as possible, then you would not even have the proportions of a dust particle.

Conclusion: In principal, an atom is practically empty. Which means in a matter of speaking, that we primarily consist of empty space!!! (And that is exactly the area in which we perform the aura surgery treatment).

And there is „something" in this masses-free space that lets us be either healthy or sick. This „something" is energy, vibes, waves or only particles, depending on if we observe it or not. And if we can bring this „something" into the right vibe, we can possibly free ourselves from illnesses.

Additional note: Our quantum physic experts recognized this nowadays after lots of thinking and research. Dr. Samuel Hahnemann, born in the year of 1755, doctor and the founder of homeopathy has already successfully implemented this 200 years ago.

Briefly deviated: Dr. Hahnemann realized the life force as he called it, determines the vibration ratio of the body. If an individual does not agree with itself or its environment, experience, and assessment, then this causes a discrepancy with the oscillating fields. The person becomes sick and needs the „dynamo gene strength of a remedy" to regulate the life principle, which is health according to Hahnemann. This is how the harmony of life is restored and the patient becomes healthy.

Dr. Samuel Hahnemann's insight: The right remedy (he called it simillimum) oscillates similar to the illness and therefore can trigger a healing reaction. To be able to heal an individual, the healthy vibration ratios have to be restored because only then a person can heal (himself). Both, physically and mentally. And even with congenital genetic defects (to this you can find more information in Dr. Prafull Vijayakar's books).

A quote from Dr. „Genius" Samuel Hahnemann: „The homeopathy can convince every thinker that the illnesses of people do not base on substances … no disease matter, but that they are the only spirit-like ones (of the life principles, the strength of life), the stimulation strength of the body of a person."

Just like aura surgery, which does „not work on substances", but on the spirit like aura.

Gisela, which you know from the foreword, is a declared fan.

GISELA, NO AGE – CATARACT

Gisela has been my patient for a few month now. Of course, you will still get to read about a mythical case of her. But today it is a complete physical diagnose that is causing her problems. The cataract makes it increasingly hard for her to see.

Let's ask Wikipedia what cataract really is: „A cataract is a clouding of the lens inside the eye. If you look at a person with advanced cataract, you can see the gray coloring behind the pupil. In most cases, the clouded lens can surgically be replaced with an artificial lens implant. The primary symptom is the slow, painless loss of the visual acuity especially when the beginning cloudiness is located in the central area of the lens. This results in a blurry eyesight and increasing sensitivity to bright light because a diffuse light refraction is generated through the cloudiness of the lens. Also, the visual perception of contrasts reduce so that the patients will see their environment „as if they see it through fog".

In the „real" cataract surgery, the cloudy, natural lens of the patient is surgically removed by an ophthalmologist and usually replaced with a so-called intraocular lens, which is made of plastic. In the circle of experts, the replacement of the natural lens is classified as the only possible treatment for a cataract.
As far as I know, this is generally the most common

surgery in Germany. Minimal invasive, short and relatively pain-free.

However, there are a few serious disadvantages that the implant shows towards the own organ. The ones that Gisela feared the most were, firstly the fact that the artificial lens could shift and a new operation would be necessary. And the second is the dependency to a good ophthalmologist because an artificial lens requires life-long checkups.

The aura surgical treatment of the clouded lens of Gisela totally differed from the surgery of a school medical working doctor. I gave Gisela the anatomy atlas and she has so to speak "personalized" the illustrated eye. Then I have, substitutional for Gisela's own lens, cleaned and rinsed the lens in the atlas. The treatment, in contrast to the surgery of a doctor, was not pain-free. Continually, Gisela had apparently felt unpleasant sensations.

As always with the quantum healing, we had a lot of help from the knowledge of the quantum field. I just allowed myself to be guided. Or as the school medicine says, I counted on the placebo effect (you will find more on the topic placebo in the next chapter).

Gisela's feedback arrived on the next day via email. I will print it here, word-for-word, unchanged and in her own staccato:

„Dear Mrs. Schlinger, because of the eyes.. it is a wonder.. on the way home I did not need sunglasses.. my eyes did not water, only a slight burning...but.. my visual acuity is not cloudy anymore.. Contours are clear.. the term that I could not remember yesterday.. the contrast acuity is now clear :-)
Usually when I got out of bed in the morning, the first

thing I did was grab my glasses,.. because I often saw everything in a blurry way.. this morning I went tot he kitchen without glasses to make me a coffee, and not until I wanted to read.. I realized that I still need them for that, but even the reading works better now ;-)

the wide angle.. it is clear again when I look to the side.. before there was always a haze.

Therefore, I can only say, thank you, I will just observe this and will inform you about the changes.

Much obliged.. I am happy… Gisela"

Up to this day, Gisela is satisfied with the performance of her eyes.

Melanie's case was not quite as easy. Her problems occurred with an injury of her eyes through a caustic ointment.

MELANIE, EARLY 20'S – TEAR IN THE CORNEA

I received the following email in January:

„Dear Mrs. Schlinger,

I have found your practice through research about aura surgery. I would like to inquire if it is possible to substantially „sew" a tear/injury in the cornea. Since my eyes have been arid for 2 years now, the surface of the eye is additionally stressed and shows symptoms of an allergy (swelling of the conjunctiva) with unknown causes.

Last week, the strained cornea of the eye has torn open again. The already healed tears open up over and over again through blinking and eye movements, so that a long-term healing success is hard to reach.

With best regards Melanie"

Melanie has been through a 2 year long treatment marathon. She has seen school medicine oriented physicists and also naturopaths. It was not easy to make an appointment for her since she was not able to travel here on her own.

When she came into my practice, her eyes were permanently hurt. Every 2-3 minutes she had to drop artificial tear fluid into her eyes to keep the pain bearable. The cause of the problem was an anti-acne ointment that had a caustic effect on the cornea of her eyes.

Melanie was very distant during the treatment. I clearly felt that she was really tense. Nevertheless, she admitted herself to this strange situation, as I gave her the anatomical atlas and asked her to give me feedback as soon as I started the treatment.

First, I substitutionally cleaned the cornea of the left eye in the atlas. Melanie was able to feel this. At the same time she let me know, that her eyes already felt less irritated. Then I rinsed the entire area of the cornea with the intention to flush out all the foreign objects that we have removed earlier. In the end, I asked god for healing tear fluid that I then let flow into the eyes.

Melanie was continually feeling better. When the treatment ended, the pain has undoubtedly eased up.

One day later I have received following email from her:
„ … The cornea of the eyes feel wonderfully smooth, especially on the left side, the intense gritty-eye sensation has also rapidly decreased and the tear film gained stability! Thank you very, very much for this! My eyes have not felt this beautiful in a long time! ;). The tear in the right eye sometimes still aches a little (blinking + eye movement), but it is not in comparison to before. …"

PLACEBO-EFFECT – YOUR METABOLISM BELIEVES IN YOU

What is the placebo effect? Firs, the definition of Planet-Wissen.de:

"Not a few alternative procedures help the patients, although it's proven that there is no effect that can come from them. Experts thereby speak of the placebo effect."

Oh man, shattering. It is proven that there is no effect. But why so they work anyways? I am asking myself firstly, who are these experts? And secondly, what are these experts for? Maybe marketing experts of the pharma industry?

But then there is still Wikipedia. According to Wikipedia, a placebo „after classical definition… is a preparation that is manufactured for medications with usual dosage form, but does not contain medically active ingredients."

 I like this definition much better. So, it is (often) a preparation, I agree to that. It does not contain medically active! Ingredients. This raises the question, what is a medication?

Because we just now received a satisfying answer, we will ask Wikipedia again: „… Medicines are developed in pharmaceutical research, where new pharmaceutical substances are identified and experimental drugs are tested in laboratory experiments and clinical studies."

Ah, so that's how it is. So, placebos are preparations that do not contain substances that were developed in pharmaceutical research and are, therefore, not protected by a registered pattern or by a patent.

And possibly inexpensive and available for free? This is a question I have that should be checked. Please check for yourself and then send me your results.

Because of the internet, actually all information's are available. We just have to find them. And we will find them if we dig deep enough!

Summarized: Placebos help the patients without having to pay taxes to the pharma industry. Am I right?!

Then let's try to find an explanation of how they work. Let's pretend as if the ingredients were information. With everything we know so far, it could actually be like that. Information's that are not developed from the pharmaceutical research. Just because they have been there all this time. So, nothing new, just old stuff. That's why there is no patentability.

Understandable? My husband always says that I should explain my brainwaves in images that are familiar to people. And he is an expert in the post automation field. There you go, honey:

We want to bring information to the destination (our patient, you). If the medication of the pharma industry were letters, which are thrown into the mailbox (mouth), which will then be emptied (swallowed) by the mailman and then they are brought to the head post office (stomach) where they are sorted (digested) and brought to a different distributor (intestinal mucosa), from where the letters are delivered by the second mailman (circulating blood) to your mailbox (target organ), where you then open and read what's in them, then the information has arrived at your cell metabolism in 1-2 days of post office running time.

If the letter was not damaged, lost or was materially damaged in any other way during the delivery. So, the medicine of the pharma industry is the letter.

And our placebo was exactly not that. It's hard to comprehend, in the literal sense. No matter, no active ingredient that is measurable. It is only information in our example. And energy. An email.
When I send it, then it is nearly simultaneous available to you.

And when the expert lurks around your mailbox for a while and waits for a letter to arrive that he could measure. Nothing will come. The information has reached you long ago.

You have probably already read it, responded to it and have informed all your friends (other organs) and tool measures to implement the information (your metabolism). And the mailman still sits outside and says: „Nothing measurable has arrived here. Nothing can take effect."

And it was really cost-effective: I have not even bought a stamp… ;-).

In the communications field, the email has replaced the letter. It's faster and cheaper. It's easier available because I don't need to get paper, envelopes, and stamps in advance, nor do I rely on the opening hours of the post office. The email is the modern medium for fast and efficient communication. In certain areas and under certain conditions, the letter still has the power, but it sure is no longer the medium of the future.

I admit that the direct comparison to the medical science is a bit far apart. But the idea is good, right?

Years ago I heard a seminar with the topic cell metabolism from Dr. Bodo Köhler in which he explains, that there are 1018 reactions per second in the call metabolism of our organism. Which are exactly 1.000.000.000.000.000.000 pieces. In every second.

Dr. Köhler also explained clearly that the psyche is the central aspect of the cell metabolism because the intention! of the cell is already being implemented. Let's assume the quantum physic again is right and has entangled quantum's that exchange their information in real-time. Then that would be a possible 1018 reactions per second because of information, right?

And now completely hypothetically: So, if I have a particular intention, e.g. to take a particular pain from my patient, then I first need the information, or the wish, the intention, or call it whatever you want. Then I need access to the cells of my patient. We already know this. Quantum entanglement. And then my information has to trigger something with the cells. That means, the cells have to read the email that contains the information. Now the intention comes into paly.

We usually read our emails. At least most of us do. But we don't read – the spam folder.

Why do we not read it? Because we „know" that it does not contain any helpful information. Just trash; maybe even worst; something that harms our system.

And how do the emails get into our spam folder? Well, through a program that runs in the background. Which we received automatically when we opened our email account.

It was free, didn't cost any extra. And the experts (see the beginning of the chapter) know what we should read or not and filter them for us.

There are sure a lot of emails that could actually harm us. Most of them we would have recognized ourselves (you have won 20 million dollars, send us your secret bank account pin and we will send you the money).
But sometimes it also filters out information that we wanted to read. The mail of a loved one, the mail of an info blog that just has too many addresses in its own or other mailing lists. But we do not even notice because we regularly, and because of lack of time, delete it.

This is also similar to how we filter the information's that reach us from the outside. Somebody is talking about mental health, quantum medicine, aura surgery. Those unheard ones land in the spam folder of our present life.

Because we have learned in our childhood that the doctor will heal us; that we are not the owner of our own body. When I am sick, I go to the doctor. He knows my body better than I do. He will give me medicine (we already know this word) so I will get healthy again.

He is also responsible for checkups. Medical checkups, immunizations (don't worry, I will not get into that), it is always an expert.

How does the doctor always know what is right for us? Because he always visits educational seminars. Where? There, where the medicine is produced, because they have developed and tested it. And are experts (we already heard this word too) for their products. And because the doctor is a specialist for our health, he is our point of contact. Because of him we "know" what works. And the rest we put aside. To the spam.

Tipp: If the quantum medicine has not (yet) worked on you, just read your spam folder. On request, you will also receive more spam from me.

We strayed away from the subject enough! Back to the aura surgery: I also have the intention to provide relief to my patients. I have found the contact to his cells, which will find out about my focused intention through the quantum entanglement. And because a person is a conglomerate to his own cells, which can communicate with each other in real-time, it can happen that the individual already feels much better during the aura surgical treatment. Like Melanie.

Or Renate.

RENATE, EARLY 60'S – CHRONIC STOMACH PAINS SINCE CHILDHOOD

Renate was in her early 60's when she came to me upon the recommendation of her sister. Since her early childhood, she has agonizing stomach pains. During the years, she had visited different doctors and went through a lot of treatments, but she never became pain-free.

The pain moves throughout her entire stomach area. In addition, she has always had problems in the area between the thoracic spine and the right shoulder.

In her childhood and also in the following years she has experienced some hard situation and traumatic incidents so that it was easy enough to push the issue onto a psychosomatic disorder.

During our aura surgery session, we have found a different cause for her organic problems. Namely, a torture and execution method that was practiced from the ancient times to the beginning of the modern times. The impalement.

Earl Vlad Tepec became famous for this execution method (1431-1477). He had a lot of his victims impaled and according to the legend, he cared to eat his meals in the middle of the tortured bodies. He received the surname „the impaler", which meant „dracul" in his language.

A sharp pole with a rounded off tip was pushed into the male victims anus, or the female victims vagina or also anus. Up to a depth of 12 inches, so the victim couldn't fall off. After that, the pole together with the victim were put up and fixated in a hole that was dug out before.

The victim suffered tremendous torments because the pole made its way through the victim's body and often pushed the vital organs to the side, which significantly prolonged the death struggle.
The pole would then emerge the body either at the neck our shoulder or between the thoracic spine and the shoulder blade.
The entire abdominal area was affected, even if the organs were not or hardly wounded. The pole was only pushed through the body weight of the victim, which took a long time most of the time, sometimes even a few days.

I lifted Renate off the pole und tended her wounds in the abdominal area, both in the aura as well as in the anatomy atlas. I felt the emerging area in Renate's aura and aura surgically closed it.

Renate told me later on that this was the exact area that she has felt the intensive pain in.

3 weeks later I received following email:

„Dear Mrs. Schlinger,
Here is the feedback for my treatment on July 24th. Since my childhood, I have had over and over occurring abdominal pain. So far, no doctor was able to help me. You lifted me off the pole and remove the post that was pushed through my body.
Ever since this moment, I have absolutely not felt any

stomach pain. It is so wonderful. I am so thankful. I want to hug you. Renate "

Dear Renate, you are welcome. But please think about that I have only given some information. You became health on your own!

MATTER – ENERGY – INFORMATION – EMOTION

Do you know the story about the truck driver that was locked into his freezer truck? He has just cleaned the cooling area as the door flew shut and the lock snapped into place. It was impossible to open the door from the inside and his colleagues already left to go home. The poor man was imprisoned and it looked as if he had to spend the entire night in his cold prison.

He was found the next day. Dead. His muscles were stiff and he showed all signs of frostbite.
Of course, you'd think. He was locked in the freezer truck for hours. But here is the remarkable thing: the freezer truck was out of use! And it was a summery day. There were no arctic temperatures in the truck for sure.

But why was the man frozen to death?

Bruce Lipton has explained it to us in his book „Intelligent Cells": The cells already react to the "intention", actually to the focus.
The truck driver surely did not have the intention to freeze to death. But his experiences let him „know", that the temperatures in the (operating) freezer truck reach double digits.
And secondly he „knew", that a person cannot survive for a very long time and will freeze to death at minus

temperatures without protection against the cold.

These two „irrevocable truths" determine his perception. All of his emotions focus on it. In his case it must have been exclusive and focused the fear of death through freezing. Because what he did not realize, because of fear, was the fact that the cooling units were out of use.

He has created his deadly reality through his focus and with the fitting emotions.

What exactly are these powerful emotions?

In the meantime, out of pure habit, we ask Wikipedia again: „The foreign word emotion names a feeling, an emotion and spiritual excitement."

That is how it was with the truck driver. In his case it was about the feeling of fear that had him and his entire consciousness concentrated on „being helplessly exposed to arctic temperatures".

Wikipedia says further: „This (the emotions) are a psychophysiological and also a psychological phenomenon that is triggered by the conscious or unconscious perception of an event or situation. The perception goes hand in hand with mental changes, particular cognitions, subjective emotional experiences and reactive social behavior. The psychophysiological deals with the relationship between the psychological processes and the underlying body functions. It describes how emotions, changes in the consciousness and behavior are connected with brain activity, circulation, respiration, motor functions and the release of hormones." (The summarized short version from Bruce: „The cells already react to the intention").

A person's body knows, how he needs to behave itself

when it is exposed to the cold.

First it will try to keep the body temperature steady. It automatically produces warmth through shivering. We all know this. In addition, the blood vessels in the arms and legs will contract to reduce the blood circulation in the outer body regions. A „bowl" develops in which the cold blood stays. The exchange of body warmth between the bowl and the core of the body almost completely stops after a while.

If a person stays in a cold environment, his consciousness will get dull more and more. It seems as if a person is asleep. Then, the reflexes will weaken and, therefore, the shivering stops. If the body temperature drops below 82.4°F, it causes a loss of consciousness, an unregulated and weakened pulse and then respiratory and cardiac arrest as a result of heart arrhythmia. Our patient dies.

Now, the crazy thing about this is: all these physical processes cannot just be caused by actual minus temperatures in the surrounding area, but only through the real fear of it. And the so created highly emotional focus, which we precisely directed to this topic.

So, death because of imagination? That's new, right?

Not really. Now, you don't have to die because of the harming information. But often enough it will just make it difficult for your body to heal. The phenomenon is known under the term „nocebo".

Exactly this happened to Roland.

ROLAND, 58 – ROOFER (AGAIN) WITH FARSIGHTEDNESS

Roland is an „accomplished craftsman". He has been leading his own roofer company for over 30 years. His wife is an excellent cook and provides him with healthy, nutrient and vitamin-rich food. He is trained and „technically" healthy through the daily physical work in the fresh air. However, he still has a physical defiance that causes a limitation for him.

In midsummer about 25 years ago he had an order for renovation work for a roof on a multi-level house. He worked all day in the blistering sun. There was no shade and he could not make up for the water loss through sweating by just drinking.

Therefore, a vein in his right eye busted. Blood ran into the surrounding tissue so that the eye was completely red. Roland was not able to see through this blood anymore.

The ophthalmologist told him that the body would get rid of the contusion on its own, however, it could take a very long time.
I will just identify this sentence as the nocebo information.

Because 25 years have passed and Roland still has to „look around" the left over streaks.

He describes it like this: „I always see thick dark threads in front of my right eye and the things I want to look at lay behind. I always have to roll and blink with my eyes so that the threads, so to speak, are pushed to the side. But after a while they back, exactly there, where they were before".

I am working in Roland's aura. I carefully feel around his eyes on all sides and I am specifically searching for the substantial area in which the contusion used to be.

In the beginning, Roland wasn't able to feel anything. But when I moved to the area where I assumed the cause for the bleeding, he noticed my touch as "furry, as if asleep". Here, about 8 inches away from his physical body, I scratched away the crust of the blood.

To not cause any more damage to the sensitive tissue, I energetically have generously flushed the entire eye with the homeopathic medication named „Arnica Montana".
Arnica is a homeopathic medication for bleeding injuries. It stops the bleeding, displays anti-inflammatory and ensures that the contusion will go away fast.

After the treatment, I asked Roland to check his vision. He had a vague feeling, as if the opaque „threads" turned lighter.

I have met him again 3 days later. He looked happy and told me that he could see much better with the treated eye. The thicker threads became much thinner and the former thin ones went away entirely. The progressive improvement continues for about 4 weeks. After that, it remained static, but the stayed in good condition.
Roland has announced that he will be back for a follow up treatment to „remove the left over threads".

GABI, 50 - DIAPHRAGMATIC HERNIA

Gabi, a vigorous 50-year-old woman, came into my practice in January. She has asked me for an appointment over the phone because she suffered the consequences of an acute diaphragmatic hernia.

Her doctor made it very clear to her that the only option to free her from the discomforts was a surgery. She was hardly able to eat and drink but, because of reasons of the organization, she had to wait a great while for a surgery appointment. This is why we made one for an aura surgical session, to decrease the level of suffering until the surgery date.

A bit of theory: the abdominal cavity and the chest cavity are separated by the diaphragm. The esophagus passes from the throat through the chest cavity and enters the abdominal cavity through a slit-like opening in the diaphragm, and then ends in the stomach shortly after. There is also a circular muscle in this spot, which prevents that the sour content of the stomach flows back into the esophagus.

Parts of the stomach can be pushed from the abdominal cavity through the slit-like opening in the diaphragm to the chest cavity above, which we then call a "diaphragmatic hernia".

And in practice: with an unbelievable effort, Gabi dragged herself into my practice on the second floor. From the beginning of the treatment, her aura clearly showed signs of an external energy. What is an external energy?

Well, it seemed as if there was another energy system besides Gabi's, bustling in her aura. In this case, it was not with evil intent, but it was probably foraging. As when we go to a sushi restaurant and take what we think looks the most delicious, the energy feasted on Gabi's strength. Increasingly in the area of her solar plexus, which, on a physical level, lies at the height of the stomach pass through her diaphragm.

First I freed Gabi from the energy and then supplied the „docking sites" in her aura. The further aura surgical operation we have performed with an anatomy atlas.

In the anatomy atlas, I freed her stomach from the embrace of the sphincter and brought the knocked up stomach parts back into the abdominal cavity. We closed the tear in the diaphragm, due to injury, with a laser and healed potential inflammations.

Gabi has changed directly after the operation in her aura, she seemed calmer, her pale face became a rosy taint and she was breathing a lot deeper.

This was also a really exciting session for me, because Gabi reacted strongly and told me exactly what and where she felt things. And the best is: during the treatment I have already felt, that as if Gabi increasingly felt better.

Gabi's personal, written report in her own words from mid-June:
„During the first week of February I went to the doctor because I was almost unable to eat and drink. Furthermore

I have felt pressure on my right side.

After I have swallowed a barium meal and my stomach was x-rayed, I was diagnosed with a diaphragmatic hernia.

A part of my stomach has pushed itself up, through a hole in the diaphragm.

I was told that this could only be corrected by surgery. …. The informational talk at the hospital made me even more uncertain. ….

On March 13th, I had my appointment for the aura surgery with Mrs. Schlinger. During the first treatment, the feeling of pressure went away. In the evening, I ate a half family pizza on my own and did not have any complaints ever since.

There should be more people that are open-minded for aura surgery. I hope a lot of people will find their way to Mrs. Schlinger.

Gabriele "

Gabriele still feels comfortable. By the way, it was shown in later x-rays that the actual physical diaphragmatic hernia did not close up. She will not delay the operation in the hospital. However, the surgery is momentarily not necessary in any way for her and doctor.

Angelika Schlinger

NOCEBO – THE IMAGINARY INVALID

You already know what a placebo is. A medication without pharmacologically active substances. „Placebo" is latin an means „I shall please" (in school, I always have been better in latin than in physics …). In 1811, the term „placebo" was first mentioned in the medical dictionary. What was meant by this was the courtesy that the doctor showed to his patients, „the discomforts that he didn't think were treatable or imagined."

The nocebo is so to say the evil brother of the placebo. The literal translation means „I shall harm".

The nocebo effect was found, when no sound effects occurred after the administration of the placebo to the patient, but negative, harmful effects. In today's medical, scientific language use, all other measures or influence quantities e.g. information's are termed as nocebo, that have no scientific-substantive prove of an effect and can cause an adverse reaction".

This is actually nothing new. This is why people of all cultures have always been scared of e.g. being cursed. The curse is „only" information. With the right curse, you could lose everything you had, become infertile, become really sick or even die.

In Germany, this phenomenon is perpetuated even in

fables; the hundred-year sleep of the sleeping beauty was more likely a rather subtle form of a curse.

The death sentences imposed by voodoo priests were examples of an extreme nocebo effect. The victims become sick and eventually actually die.

So, is the nocebo effect an imaginary sickness that possibly results in death? Of course. Because – right: the energy follows the attention! And everything we create, we think firstly. And then it can become material. An example?

If you want to build a chair, what do you do? First you will think about was you actually want. At this point, you don't even need to know what that thing is going to be called. You just want something you can sit on. So it needs a surface to sit on. It should be comfortable. Cushions would be a solution. Andi t would be nice to lay back. For this, it needs a backrest. And so you can put that thing into a different room, it should not be bound to one spot. So, a light material would be advantageous. Thought, imagined, focused, got the material and built. This and no other way is how a chair is created. The thought is the father of the chair. But that's not all.

Our ancestors knew it: „The wish is the father of the thought". Only the emotions make the thought to a reality. The wish in a positive and the fear in a negative sense.

The thought is also the father of physical changes. If you go into resonance with information (energy), or if you build up a similar oscillation with your mind, and therefore in your body, then matching changes can be materialized.

What do you think, how far can this go? Is suicide through a nocebo possible?

I don't know. But there is this case that is described by Roy R. Reeves in the Journal „General Hospital Psychiatry" (2010).

A student wanted to end his life and took a whole month's supply of medication that he received through the participation in a medicine study. His condition was very critical, so he had to undergo a medical treatment. The medication he took were placebo pills but since this was a blind study, he did not know. Only when he found out about the real consistency of the tablets his values normalized.

Did the young man go into resonance with the „knowledge" of the (side) effects of real medicine? Is this possible in such severe form? And if so, should one even read the package leaflet of his medicine? Should one be informed of the risks before the surgery? And if not, how would you decide things? More and more questions.

A short summary of the thoughts on nocebo:

The idea of a physical injury is the forefather of the illness. Providing that you „know" the effects of the substance and that you go into resonance with that. For me as an aura surgeon it is thereby insignificant, if the consciousness of the patient knows about the material consistency of a substance or if „only" the unconsciousness goes into resonance.

You already know: quantum entanglement, information exchange in real time, emotion to that, energy follows the attention, matter follows the energy… A physical symptom is made. Whether a chair, tumor or incidentally the free parking space, everything is possible.

That's what the modern science says. And the aura surgery too. Wonderful, we're keep getting closer.

KERSTIN, 42 – BENDY LEG CORRECTION „WITHOUT THE LOWER LEG"

It was spring when Kerstin came to me. Since her childhood she suffered from massive bendy legs, which resulted in a painful arthrosis in both knee joints.

A couple of years ago she went to her trusted orthopedist and had undergone a surgery on her right knee. A so-called sled, a knee replacement, was inserted. The surgery went very well. Since years, Kerstin was a finally able to walk relatively pain-free with her right leg, she was very satisfied with the result.

A couple of months ago, she then had the second knee operated on with the same procedure. For the second time, the risks of the operation were told to her. Can you already guess what happened?

Anyway, Kerstin (deliberately) expected the same good results because her left knee that was somewhat less worn out, less arthritic and less painful. She was entirely wrong.
The recovery after the second surgery considerably dragged on. Even weeks after the straightening the knee stayed swollen, inflamed and painful.

When Kerstin came to see me, her right knee was slightly swollen and slightly painful. Her left knee was as big as her thigh, hot, inflamed and painful.

We first treated her right leg with the aura surgery. The operation was not just a success on her physical body, even in her aura it seemed to have left behind a wonderful result. Obviously there was only some energetic synovial fluid missing that is why there was an inflamed area. Kerstin was very sensitive. We filled energetic synovial fluid into it, which she experienced as calming. To test the effect, she walked back and forth in the treatment room. The knee felt „softer", like i fit was well lubricated. Kerstin was satisfied.

After that, I tested her left knee. Also here, Kerstin was really sensitive above her knee joint. In her aura, I felt the area of her thigh that connects to her knee joint. Kerstin experiences this as unpleasant, almost painful. The area of the fake knee joint didn't feel natural to me, but it also didn't feel disturbing. Apparently, Kerstin's surgeon has placed the metal sled into her biological system so that it was even accepted by her energy body. However, the inflammation was massive, the knee swollen and it seemed as if her body did not want accept the knee replacement.

I felt along her leg and further down into the area of the lower leg in Kerstin's aura. Suddenly Kerstin was not able to feel anything anymore. And I was not able to feel anything either. It was as if there was no lower leg at all.

From her point of view, Kerstin confirmed the exact same feeling. The image of an accident victim with an amputated left lower leg forced itself upon me. So I energetically asked for a new lower leg, took it with joy and gratitude and connected the new energy with the one of the amputation limb.

Kerstin did not feel well during this procedure. She was

really pale and her pulse raced. As fast as I could I adjusted the energetic connection of the knee and lower leg, stitched it and closed it with a laser. All vessels and nerve tracts in the energy field were connected again as Gerhard Klügl taught us. Kerstin felt better more and more. She sat for a while and collected herself. After that, I could let her leave to go home
.

A few days later, she thanked me via email. She literally wrote: „I would be delighted to be mentioned in your book. After all, you were the one who accomplished that I can again stand in life with both feet. Kind regards, Kerstin."

Angelika Schlinger

KERSTIN SUBSEQUENT TREATMENT – FINALLY TAKING A PART IN LIFE

In a bit, I will let Kerstin speak for herself. A couple of days after her subsequent treatment, we carried out the routine phone conversation to discuss any changes.

Shortly after, I received this email from her:

„Hello, Frau Schlinger!
I have sat down immediately to write the story of my bladder. I call it "Finally, taking a part in life again, I am back again!"

In the beginning, my bladder problems were only a minor matter until I didn't feel comfortable anymore.

Everything started with the knee surgery I had undergone in February. It was the same surgery I had a year ago, only more painful and that is why I had to use my bladder catheter for longer than planned. When I was finally able to get up and stand, it was removed. Ever since there has been blood in my urine.

Three weeks of rehabilitation followed for my knee. During my final examination, I have mentioned my bladder and also the increased urge to urinate and the massive red outflow.
The doctor said that the bladder wall was wounded

when the catheter was removed and that my family physician should give me some antibiotics. However, since I still had intense pain in both knees at the time and still took strong pain killers, I was not willing to swallow antibiotics on top of that.

My nerves were completely on the edge, and my bladder was only a minor matter to me at the moment.

Because I have already seen Mrs. Schlinger at this point because of my operated knee and she has helped me to be able to normally walk and also helped me with the movement of my legs, I asked her for advice about my bladder.

I explained the urgency to urinate and the orange-red urine to her. I sat on a chair in front of her and she grabbed a book (an anatomy atlas, in which a picture of a bladder was illustrated) and with a scalpel she cut along the bladder.

She said that my bladder mucosa was injured. With a syringe, she injected a fluid into my bladder so that the bladder walls were coated. I felt how the bladder was filling up. There was a pressure, there was something warm, and it felt as if I had to go to the bathroom. When I went to the bathroom at home, the urine was almost clear and when I went a second time it was clear and colorless.

Everything was good for one week and then it started all over again. I was at a loss and disappointed. I had the urge to urinate again for two weeks and hat to use pantyliners to not dirty all of my underwear. What happened?

I asked Mrs. Schlinger during the next appointment. She explained to me that all my cells had fallen back into their old scheme and have to be reminded again that there is something new. We then have coated the bladder mucosa with fluid again. I too felt this time, how the bladder filled up, it was pressure, not painful but not unpleasant either.

At home I immediately went to the bathroom and Thank God, everything was fine again! I felt like a new woman and as a reward I went to the open public pool.

I haven't been to the pool in 2 years because I could not even walk a short distance with my bad knee. I was swimming for 25 minutes and I felt great, my legs did not hurt anymore and the best thing was, I did not have to be scared of dirtying my swimsuit because of my bladder weakness. THANK YOU !!!!!

So, Mrs. Schlinger, my story became a little longer. You can shorten it and of course you can use my full name. Kerstin Uhlendorf"

Dear Mrs. Uhlendorf that is an incredible story. Of course, I will not shorten it.

WHEN DIAGNONES KILL

„Urologists possibly need to be more gentle when diagnosing prostate cancer: Just two days after receiving the bad message, affected people noticeably often decide for suicide – or suffer a deadly heart attack within one year."

You can read the original text online on news.doccheck.com. On top, you can find the entire article under the title: "When Diagnoses Kill".

It further says, that a few only days or month after the diagnose of prostate cancer, men „sometimes decide for suicide or die because of a heart attack as a result of the enormous burdens, as a current study of the „Journal of the National Cancer Institute" attested."

According to the article, a survey based on more than 340.000 patient's information from 1987 to 2004 of the American cancer registry has been implemented at the Boston Harvard Medical School under the leadership of Fang. So this is a big study with valid numbers and not just some small, short mini-study.

To Fang's surprise, 6.845 men died from a heart attack, primarily within the first three months after the diagnosis, 148 prostate cancer patients committed suicide. (After everything we know, it wasn't going to surprise us, right?)

I particularly find the numbers of the heart attack impressive. When a person decides on suicide then, it is a decision he consciously makes for himself at that moment. A heart attack is a decision of the body, without asking its owner. (Well, he has probably pointed it out a few times that it is in a sorry state. The person did not listen.)

Now there is the diagnosis „cancer" - and the person immediately becomes a patient with a (he has learned that) deadly diagnose. The intense fear emotion is added to that. The person goes into resonance with death. And since we get what we create energetically, the deadly heart attack will come.

With this theory, I am probably heavily competing with the numerous diagnose- and therapy forms that would name the heavy mental burden as a reason for the heart attack.

The psycology calls this somatization. Somatization describes „tendency, physical indisposition and symptoms that are not attributed to pathological organic findings, ascribed to a physical illnesses and strive for a medical treatment.
It is anticipated that this tendency is often a reaction to psychosocial burdens. Other authors describe that the persisting somatization ("somatic fixation") can also play a role in organic illnesses."

But how does the implementation of the psycho- or psychosocial burden to physical symptoms like a heart attack work? Maybe through the focus on dying? Resonance? Vibe? Quantum entanglement? Maybe.

Oh, I have an interesting thought: When women are prompted to permanently check their breasts for knots and to regularly go to the mammography, then they also have a particular focus. And that is not just intellectually, but also physically implement. Brain and hand are looking for a knot.

By the way, our brain doesn't like it, when it searches for a solution but isn't able to find one. It searched for a knot, it searches and searches – until one day the resonance is finally there and our brain finally finds what it was looking for. The brain thinks: „Ah, there you go!" … Has anyone ever thought about this side of the precaution health examination?

But what does the word precaution mean? Well, actually: To be worried about something before, right? To go into massive resonance with the fear emotion? A self-fulfilling prophesy? Or is this too philosophical for you? Are there studies on this topic? If there is a reader out there with information about this, I would like to talk about it. You can find my email address at the end of the book.

Angelika Schlinger

INVESTIGATED – A HEART ATTACK IS NO CANCER

What did you say? You want to go back to the topic. And you think that a heart attack and cancer are two different things? Yes, for now, you are right.

But the fact is that we have to tell the quantum field exactly what we want to have. Or we get the manifestation that we specifically „think here" with our most intensive emotions. The more precise and more specific we define it the more likely we get exactly what we wish for. Or in the opposite, we are scared of.

The physicists call it the zero-point field (quantum field). The zero-point field is the source of all beings and all realities – basically it is the source of all that exists. It is the state before an object materializes or before a situation occurs. It is, so to say, the (time-) space between 2 thoughts.

Frank Kinslow identifies it as the space, from where your next thought will come. In the zero-point field, all possible realities are present. Whichever one actually turns up, manifests itself, whichever one you choose for yourself, that is your decision. And as said, the more precisely you define for yourself on what your reality should look like, the closer your implementation will be to your personal goals.

FASCINATION AURA SURGERY

Albert Einstein said the field is the only reality. After that comes the actuality that you create for yourself. And this is how it works:

You wish for more money. And you really want it with a lot of emotions because you just have too little money. And then you realize: the money is laying in the street. In the form of a 5 cent piece. Great, says the quantum field, he wanted more money and he promptly received it. Super. And you are still dissatisfied. Instead of being thankful that your wish immediately came true, you are still on the look-out, doubting the existence of a wish-fulfilling-machine in the quantum field.

It is not entirely unlikely to run into money just through wishing?! And your doubts turn into certainty. Of course, because – right, always the same consequence: the energy follows the attention. And your next thought has already become reality: there is no more money.

Or you create a different reality out of the zero-point field. If there really are all opportunities in it, you could make it more precise. Set yourself a real goal. A timeframe and a measurable result are counted among a goal. So not: I wish for more money. But: Today next year, I will have 100.000 Euro in my checking account of my house bank and are otherwise entirely debt free. And then you imagine with all you feelings and enthusiasm how it feels, how the ice cold champagne tastes that you're drinking to mark the occasion with your loved ones, how you sit at the beach/in your favorite bar/on your terrace and read your bank statement from which 100.000 Euro are shining towards you in black numbers…

And so on; You know what I was driving at. Do that every morning after getting up and every evening before going to bed. And in between, don't just lay around on your sofa and watch private commercial stations, but pursue the hints, tips and call to action that the quantum field sends you!! You need to act!

This zero-point field or quantum field, where is it anyways? It is with you, around you, inside you, inside me and everywhere else.

Do you remember Prof. Dr. Markolf Niemz in his book „Lucy with a c"? He explains the following:
"As seen from earth, time elapses for everything that does not travel with the speed of light. Consequently, also for the soul that spreads with the speed of light. ... The theology has characterized one term that precisely describes this state: Eternity."

So, when something spreads with the speed of light, which is literally eternally long, then I don't see the possibility, that it's not actually everywhere. So, the immortal soul is literally ubiquitous, everywhere and always! And because the quantum field is in everything, it is also in our immortal soul - voila, the quantum field just had to be everywhere.

So there are no excuses anymore. „I couldn't do it the like I actually wanted to, I had no signal", at the most, you can only use such excuses when sending an email. The quantum field, however, is always reachable!

But you also have to use it correctly. The quantum field does not grade, we've seen this with the 5-cent-piece-reality. It also does not differentiate what you rate as positive or negative. It gives you what you create, by attaching your beliefs and emotion to it.

And with that: back to the heart attack... and to cancer! If a person slips into the role of a cancer patient thoughts and fears in a patient will arise like lightning because of the diagnosis. At first the fears will be just as unspecific as the wish for money in the 5-cent-piece-realtity was. Although, the wish „I would like more money" was fulfilled with the 5 cent piece, the hoped for details (a lot of money, 100.000 Euro) were not implemented.

It is similar to the fears of our patient. The big fear of the fatal outcome of the illness was promptly implemented, but not the details of the prostate cancer symptoms.

So when you say: „A heart attack and cancer are two entirely different things", then the quantum medical answer to this can only be a „Yes, but…"!

Angelika Schlinger

DISTANT HEALING – QUANTUM ENTANGLEMENT IN ACTION

The probably most popular German Christian healer Bruno Gröning (1906 - 1959) did it, and also Harry Edwards (1893 – 1976) the spiritual Englishman, and also modern healers do it such as the Spanish physicist Alvaro Polo or the Japanese Harumi Koyama.

I am talking about distant healing. In England and Switzerland, healers with this technique are already used as co-therapists by doctors and hospitals. In Germany, they are still declined with incomprehension and skepticism.

But really: I love distant healing. They are so easy, pain-free, usable at all times and always available. It does not matter where you are. It does not matter where I am. It's the Rolls Royce of the Placebos ;-).

Why do they work? There are probably a lot of answers. I stick with the quantum physics. Or with the early Christian teachings because I am convinced that they both say the exact same thing. The topic distant healing is „just" practiced quantum entanglement:

You remember: Two particles meet at some point on their trip, exchange information and even when they part again on different ways, they will stay in contact the entire time. Thereby, the particles will exchange their conditions and, therefore, their information. In real-time (synchronicity). Everything is connected to everything.

If that's how it is, then the distant healing is only a logical consequence. That's what I think. And therefore I just do it. And that's the result:

Angelika Schlinger

DR. JUR. ERNST PECHTL – DISTANT HEALING LUMBAR SPINE

„Dear Mrs. Schlinger,
For a few years, I have been suffering from problems with the intervertebral discs in the lumbar spine area. Because of the recommendation of the doctors, I already have had a booked surgery date. However, I have canceled it in the hope to find another solution for the impairment of the right leg and pain.

At the beginning of June, the pain became a real problem especially when laying down, I had permanent pain and couldn't turn around anymore.

This was unbearable and that is why I have contacted you for help on June 9th by phone. You have then treated me from over 90 miles away.

Three days later, on the morning of June 12th I was surprised by your text message with the question: "Good morning, how are the neuralgias in the leg?? Better?"

I answered: "No, not better, they just completely went away!

6 weeks have passed since then and I have not had any pain while laying down.

This kind of was hard to imagine, because I have never experienced it before nor have I heard of it from other people!

This is how it ideally should be! At this point, I would like to express my thanks and admiration. Also, I can generally only feel small „leftovers" of the problem with

intervertebral discs, especially when sitting in bad chairs. But I am confident that you can wangle that too…
Best regards,
Dr. jur. Ernst Pechtl, Dipl.-Kfm.
Verona, Italy, August 21st"

Dr. jur. E. Pechtl has expressly authorized me to print his case with his name. I am stoked, because a doctor in law is a candidate to take seriously, even for the big skeptics out there.

Or is anyone questioning this?

Angelika Schlinger

KATRIN, 50 – TENNIS INSTEAD OF ARM SLING

I have known Katrin, who's also a therapist as a patient from an aura surgical session "on site". She was interested in this form of therapy and booked an aura surgical treatment in my practice to feel the effect on her own body. That was at the beginning of June.

We then spoke on the phone a couple of days later to talk about her experiences and to clarify possible questions.

Thereby she told me about another problem with her right elbow. It felt wounded, inflamed und hurt severely as soon as she stressed it. Sports performances were undoable. As a tennis player, she was really concerned, especially since I wanted to make her available for a match a few days later.

We were unable to place an appointment in the practice, so I offered her to do distant healing. Katrin agreed. (What other choice did she have).

For the distant healing, I use a replacement for the physical patient. Favorably a good anatomy atlas, in which all body parts and organs are illustrated in detail.

For Katrin's elbow, I found an illustration of all layers,

from bones and joints to tendons, muscles, nerves up to the skin.

From the beginning, I casted suspicion on the tendons as the cause of Katrin's pain. For the aura surgical distance healing, I have worked myself inside out beginning at the joints.

Different muscle groups have their roots in the area of the elbow. They are all grown together with the elbow bone through tendons made of connective tissue.
If you consciously tighten and then extend your forearm, you will realize that different muscle groups, and thereby also different tendons, are responsible for the bending and stretching.
It is bent, who would be surprised, with the arm bender biceps that run along on the inside of the elbow. The opponent is the arm stretcher triceps, which is located on the outside.
Through the over-stressing of the muscle group, a so called epicondylitis humeri can occur. A syndrome with the ending –itis is always in inflammation. The epicondylitis is also a paraphrased inflamed pain syndrome in the elbow area.

In Katrin's case it was, according to the information of her quantum entanglement tested, a tennis elbow. It is an inflamed, due to wear scar tissue directly by the bone that causes the pain.

The school medicine treats the tennis elbow mostly conservatively, which means, at first without surgery. Rest is the most important thing. Then physiotherapy with special stretching exercises, shock wave therapy and bandages. Really time-consuming.

We didn't have time, because Katrin didn't want to rest

her arm, she wanted to play the important match. So I was looking for a faster solution.

I checked Katrin's tendons in the anatomy atlas. The starting points of the tendons, and also in the bone area, seemed overstrained; they felt hot, swollen and sensitive.

I energetically asked for a remedy that relieves the pain, reduces the inflammation and that puts the body in a position, for it to reduce scar tissue. I have drawn this solution into a syringe and slowly injected it into the aura of the areas that need to be treated.

After a half hour, the treatment was finished. That was on Thursday.
The tennis match was going to take place on the following Saturday.

And on Sunday I have received following email from Katrin:

„Subject: Tennis
Hello Angelika,
I kept up pretty good in the game!!! It was painful, but the elbow didn't feel as sore and vulnerable, and that's the most important thing. I lost because I primarily had splendid opponents. Again, thank you so much and I wish you all the best Katrin"

By the way: Katrin has pharmaceutical training and medical knowledge. So she knows, that all illnesses should be taken seriously. She would never act negligently and never renounce the diagnosis of a doctor or naturopath for a questionable therapy. I hope, you treat your body just as responsible!

HOW MANY TIMES? – ALWAYS REBIRTH

At the beginning of Christianity the rebirth, the reincarnation was an inherent part of the belief. Early church dignitaries and theologists like Origenes, Basilides or the saint Gregory naturally taught the re-embodiment of the soul.

An individual eventually has to develop itself, life isn't enough to get to know all sides of being. Hunger and abundance, victim and offender, man and woman, good and evil, and so on.

Even the Hinduism and its „daughter-religion", the Buddhism, know the rebirth.
The ancient Greek, from Pythagoras to Platon, were also sure of it.

One of the today's well-known representative of this certainty is Professor Ian Stevenson (1918 -2007), a Canadian psychiatrist and founder of the reincarnation research. Stevenson caused an international stir with his researches. In almost 40 years he has documented a total of 2.600 cases, in which people told him about their former lives.

Especially the reports from children seemed believable to me, because they spontaneously, without hypnosis, reported about the memories of their previous lives. Prof. Stevenson found out that about half of the people from his study have died a violent death in their previous life. Maybe these particular souls, who didn't expect their lives to end like that, remember their past life more often.

Thereby, the victims often suffer corresponding injuries. In a lot of cases, the physical traces of such injuries occur again in the new life - in the form of scars, malformation, and moles.

You remember Peter, the easy-rider-entrepreneur with the tear in his lung?!

Mental memories, such as the fear of height, deep water or similar ones or also the dislike of particular countries (like Christine and her experience with the electric chair), can also be transferred into the next life.

So I am in good company when I am confident that these old patterns and injuries can be healed and such physical and mental problems can be eliminated with the help of aura surgery.

Anyway, Karin is confident of it.

KARIN, 45 – DIED FOR THE SCOTTISH CLAN: ONLY WHO KNOWS THE RULES CAN REALLY PLAY

Karin came to me because she was, from the earliest childhood on, the "leper child" in her family. Her sister was and is mommy's favorite and her brother was the favorite child of the now decedent father.

Karin was the buffer of the aggressiveness of both parents. Since she has been treated badly from early childhood on, she could not even make out a conscious „offense" on her side that could have justified the behavior of her parents. She did not only suffer from the withdrawal of affection and physical abuse. She only received absolutely essential material contributions.

In addition, she was imposed to take the responsibility, which she actually tried to carry, for the wellbeing of the entire rest of the family. Despite better conscious knowledge, she still falls back to this massive formative pattern.

For quite a while, Karin has been spending time with her familiar situation and its impact. The trigger for her aura surgery appointment with me was the current fact that she was going to be decisively disadvantaged (again) in the inherit decisions of her mother. A situation that was considered as entirely natural by her mom and sister.

Karin explains her situation like this:

„I came to Angelika's aura surgery because of the everlasting accusations and discrimination of my family towards me.

In the beginning, the felt around my aura. At first it clearly showed "old memories" of a life in Scotland. That was really interesting because, through a lot of traveling, Scotland is really familiar to me; I feel as if it was my „actual" home. I was born and raised in Germany.

With a naturopath, I have already worked on the next symptom that showed: my constant „ice legs". Most of the time my legs, from the knees to the feet, feel as if they were stuck in ice water. This sensation was strongly present again at that moment.

I have known for a while that I have lived in Scotland in the 17th century. Back then in the middle of winter, my village was attacked by English soldiers, the entire place was supposed to be wiped out. I survived. Then I have died of the consequences of the escape.

At first Angelika treated my frozen legs.
The current problem with my family was not even mentioned yet. Emotionally it was clear, that I have known my today's family members from a previous life.

During the aura surgical treatment, high emotions were released in me. Then I felt the surety that I was a clan leader back then. And despair aroused in me, because of my death I have abandoned my family and my people.

And suddenly the realization, that in fact I have been held a prisoner of war by my present family and I am still treated like this today, as if I had to be infinitely thankful for ever crumb that's thrown at me, and always have to be available when my mother needs me. So to say, I apparently have been growing up as a Scot und in an English family.

To be honest, the sudden realization was a shock to me at first. Angelika has treated not only my physical wound with the aura surgery, but also my spiritual ones. That has helped me a lot.

When I think about it, the session has not just revealed the game rules of the previous life and what running in the background of my present family, but it has opened the next door and I have discovered new rules that (maybe) only concern this life but run hand in hand with the previous life in Scotland. Today's occurrences within my family are anything but satisfying, but now I can lean back and wait.

It is so fantastical and crazy. It is as if the blindfold was removed from my eyes and I can see more every day. The behavior of my mother and sister are still hard to digest for me. But is nothing in comparison to what life, with this constellation, has brought me so far."

I want to thank Karin for being so open. Because I know that the process was receiving for her, because so far she had questioned her whole personality because of the experiences of her childhood and youth.

To bolster up people takes a lot of strengths, especially in her case. The power of a leading personality.

Angelika Schlinger

MARY, MID 50'S – I FEEL CHANGED

Mary, a cultivated, attractive woman in her mid-50's came to my practice upon the recommendation of her friend. During the admission of her case she told me that she has been to multiple examinations of different specialists.

She has not been told a confirmed cause of her problems. The diagnoses varied between fibromyalgia and psychosomatic pain.

This is how she describes the situation: „I felt horrible in the last few months. Physical pain, no energy! I am usually a positive person, but I completely secluded myself. I just didn't see a way for my future."

When I tested her aura, everything felt kind of the same. There were no clear blockages. However, there was also no strength and tension.

I asked Mary, what spontaneously comes to her mind if I wanted to know how she felt right now. Without thinking about it, she answered: „I feel changed".

The breaking wheel was a cruel way of execution up until the early 19th century in Germany and France, whereby the delinquent's bones, or the joints, on arms, legs and shanks were broken with a dissected wheel (protruded iron part).

In France, this took place with an iron rod (bar). After, the individuals that were often still alive, were „braded" onto a cartwheel and were left die (see redensarten-index.de).

I had to delete the memento of this ordeal out of Mary's cellular memory. So I took her off the wheel and aligned her joints, repaired the broken bones and healed her inner organs in the aura. After, I have newly aligned her utterly crushed spine to its full extent.

I suggested her, to lay down and to rest after the treatment because of experience, such extensive restoration is exhausting to the energy body.

This is what Mary wrote in her email, word for word:
„ Hello, Mrs. Schlinger, I could understand the recognition of the „being changed" right away. After my appointment with you, I was totally tired and exhausted, even on the next day.
My entire body feels a relief, the tensions, and the pain have resolved. (I have not felt this good in a long time.) Only the left knee and left side (torso) do not feel entirely good.
When I talked on the phone with my daughter after the appointment, she said to me: You are really different in the past weeks, more positive, a whole another voice.
Thank you! Kind regards from Mary."

Angelika Schlinger

„THE ARGUMENT, LIVING ORGANISMS ARE ONLY ELPAINABLE THROUGH THE LAWS OF PHYSICS AND THE VITALITY OF POWER DOES NOT EXIST, DOES NOT CORRESPOND WITH THE MODERN QUANTUM THEORY."

This is not a wisdom from me, but a quote from Werner Karl Heisenberg that you can read in „Quantum Philosophy and Spirituality" by Ulrich Warnke.

And this knowledge isn't entirely new either; already in 1932, Mr. Heisenberg has received the Nobel Prize in physics for his work. And he died in 1976, so almost 40 years ago.

So, if we roughly estimate, then this information is known for a good 80-100 years in the expert groups of physics.

Later on, it then has also gotten around to non-physicists.

But sadly, it has not gotten around to our secondary schools. That is at least my subjective impression. My son and my daughter have taken their Abitur in different schools, both successfully. And this information was not thought to them in class.

FASCINATION AURA SURGERY

If you are a student in the upper secondary or if you know one that has gotten this information in physics class, please send me an email as soon as possible with the name and location of the school. I will provide a written pardon. You already know, you can find my contact information at the end of the book.

Back to the topic: the scientists develop new things, so the mankind can benefit from it. (I will just assume this, so I can build my thesis on it).

So why should we, 80 years later, be content with the pure material medicine? Since we know, for about three or even four generations now, that it is just a part of the solution?

I want to get back to my example of the communication area. We are back to the letter. 80 years ago there was paper and ink, ballpoint pens were patent pending. However, they were not yet manufactured. Only in 1945, the first ballpoint pen was produced in series. This was 13 (thirteen!) years after Mr. Heisenberg received his Nobel Prize.

40 years later, there was the email. In Germany, the first internet email was received on August 3rd, 1984 at 10:14 AM MEZ. From Michael Rotert from the University of Karlsruhe.

And now I'm asking you: How many people still work with a fountain pen and a sheet of paper? And in comparison to that, how many individuals use emails to communicate? Or a text message or WhatsApp and they appeared even later!

Now it is really the time to put on new media, not only in the field of economic communication.

We should also raise the communication of our body cells with the rest of the world, with the universe to a new level. Because one thing is clear: All old religions and the modern scientific knowledge of the quantum physics agree: Our consciousness creates our reality. Our experiences steer our thoughts.

And thereby, our emotions are the catalyst.

THE LAW OF RESONANCE OR – MONEY MAKES MONEY

Another relevant law of the quantum world: The same attracts the same. The law of resonance.

That means nothing but, that we send out something that then rings back to us in unison (in Latin re-sonare means re-sounds; Yeah, learned something again). And increases itself. Because whatever you lay for focus on, will automatically draw more of it.

And because the quantum field does not grade, you will always get more of what you lay your focus on. It does not matter if you personally classify it as positive or negative.

That's why you should think about if you should constantly get angry at your uncomprehending husband, your jealous wife, your unfair boss or your mobbing neighbor. Or if you should talk about your ailments or should occupy yourself with the details of incurable illnesses on the internet. Or if you should be scared of unemployment and being broke every day.

Or if you wake up in the morning and look forward to a healthy, happy, successful day. Full of harmony, energy and sunny hours. Full of inner and outer wealth. Because if you create your own reality, it includes your health and a lot more. Your surroundings, the people you are surrounded by and also your bank account.

My dad has always pragmatically said it like this: „Money makes money".

When I was about to get my driver's license at the age of 18, a car dealer in my hometown held a raffle for a brand new Golf. It „was clear" to me that I will definitely not have money to buy a car as high-school graduate. Especially not a new one. I „knew" this for sure. Because I was broke, as a student should be… A different person in this town was a wealthy entrepreneur. He drove big BMW, his wife a Porsche. We both were present for the raffle of the new Golf, we both have bought a raffle ticket for 50 Pfennig each – and you can guess who won.
(If you do not know the answer, send me an email to faszination.aurachirurgie@mail.com, I will then reveal it to you).

Today I would have a bigger chance to win a car. Because I have learned from the aura surgery, that when I focus on a solution, I can create exactly this solution. Thereby it is not important, how this goal is achieved. Just that it is achieved. In love, harmony, and gratefulness. It is really easy. You just have to do it.

Like Gerda.

GERDA, 49 – SINGLE MOM RIPE FOR A VACATION

Gerda saw me in my practice because of muscle tension in her neck and tinnitus. She is a single mom of a 14-year-old daughter and an 8-year-old son. 3 years ago, Gerda was divorced in a not so friendly way. Meanwhile, the contact to her ex-husband is back on a tolerable level because the son has a good a relationship with his father and the parents have to exchange themselves regularly.

Gerda works full time as a geriatric nurse. She likes her job, even though it is exhausting and the pay is low.

We have solved the causes of Gerda's muscle tension and tinnitus problem in an aura surgery session. Not until afterward it showed, that Gerda had a much bigger problem.

She was utterly exhausted. The hard job, the responsibility of the two children, constantly being there for others had physically and mentally brought her to her limits. Gerda was in desperate need of a time-out.

She did not want to apply for a cure. She said: „I do want to get away. But I don't wish to sit in discussion groups with burnout- and depressed patients. That just puts me down even more."
And she did not have the needed money for a vacation.

„I don't even want to think about a vacation. I can't afford it anyways. I have thought about it a lot, but I just don't have the money". You probably notice the parallel to the Golf raffle!

We have spoken about the law of resonance. I have asked her to imagine her vacation, in the way she would define it ideal for herself. Gerda was not very demanding.

A couple of days of "girl's vacation" with her daughter were enough for her. Her son should be well-taken care of so that she could relax without a guilty conscience towards him. Then I asked her to endorse into the feeling as if she was already enjoying her vacation. Deeply relaxed, calm, refreshed, happy and whatever else she felt with it. I let her go home with this feeling.

She called me 2 days later. Her ex-husband has picked up their son on the weekend. And, he urgently wanted to talk to her. An order, which Gerda has collected for the business before their divorce, came up late (after over 3 years). The customer had paid his bill. And her ex-husband wanted to be fair towards her and brought her 1.200 Euro as a commission.

Gerda booked a week of wellness vacation with her daughter while her son could spend a father-son adventure week with his dad.

THE CIRCLE CLOSES – OFF TO NEW WATERS

As you see, the aura surgery has brought a lot of zest into my everyday practice life and into the lives of my patients. So, some questions have been answered, a few knots have been undone and a lot has changed to the positive.

3 weeks ago, Brigitte Kellermann has held an aura surgery meeting for Gerhard Klügl in an out of the way hotel. Far away from any civilization we were able to exchange experiences, pass on tips and tricks and spend an exciting, entertaining and once again an educational weekend together in a circle of colleagues. Mutual aura surgical treatment included because as a therapist you rarely get a chance for an own aura surgery session.

How it always is: not only the professional lectures lead to new knowledge. Especially the personal talks during the „lecture free time" create new impulses and ideas. And that is how new approaches for the use of aura surgery have extracted for me. In the following weeks, I will overthink and structure them. And develop a new project for sure. I wonder what topic that will be.

If you want to be involved, if you want to co-design, if you have suggestions or also new, fresh ideas – then you are welcome to participate! Visit my new web page www.faszinationaurachirurgie.com and I will introduce you.

I will show you the approaches and will report to you about the current state of the project. Your opinion can be significant for the development. I will pull some strings and will introduce Brigitte Kellermann to you, my savior from the first seminar, and will send you her contact information, if she says yes... And there, you might also find the address of a qualified aura surgeon in your surrounding area.

Because you should not miss the chance of your on aura surgery session. Either in apractise or as a distance healing.

CONTACT AND EXCHANGE OF IDEAS

Are you too fascinated from the aura surgery? Or do you have questions or suggestions? Do you even have improvement suggestions for my book?

Then send me an email right away to

faszination.aurachirurgie@gmail.com

I can't wait to read your opinions and thoughts.

If you liked the book, then it would be a pleasure to receive a review on Amazon. Thank you!

THANK YOU

To everyone that has helped with the development of this book.

Thank you Gerhard Klügl, for the training, foreword and the humor that makes you so unique.

Thank you to my husband Gregor for his open ear, critical notes, and constant proofreading that let me find the right way over and over again.

A special thank you to my mother. The proofreading was probably not easy for you because I know, that the topic is really „spacey" to you.

Thanks to my dad for the understanding of the devil's digestion logic.

Thank you to all my kids, Alexander, Johanna and also Shaki, that added their two cents.

Thank you to Dr. Eleonore Blaurock-Busch, the scientist and uncrowned laboratory queen of toxic analysis. When you give your OK to the publishing, then rest of the scientists can kiss ... and Mail me of course, for any questions!

And thank you Pamy, whom I lost sight of for such

long time and still has made herself available as a lecturer in the last minute.

And last not least thank you Stefanie Colbert for your wonderful translation.

And a sincere thank you to you, dear readers. It was a pleasure to spend your reading time with you.

I have really hit the jackpot with all of you.

BIBLIOGRAPHY

1. Werner Heisenberg in Ulrich Warnke: Quantenphilosophie und Spiritualität. Scorpio, 2011

2. Gerhard Klügl: Quantenland: Ein Leben als Aurachirurg. Arkana, 2012

3. Bruce Lipton: Intelligente Zellen: Wie Erfahrungen unsere Gene steuern. Koha Verlag, 2013

4. Markolf H. Niemz: Lucy mit c: Mit Lichtgeschwindigkeit ins Jenseits. Books on Demand, 2006

5. www.wikipedia.de

ABOUT THE AUTHOR

Angelika Schlinger has been working as a naturopath in her own practice for over 20 years (www.praxis-schlinger.de). Next to her consolidated training in the classical homeopathy, she uses her knowledge and experiences, in the field of clinical metal toxicology, for the treatments mostly of chronic illnesses. She describes her enthusiasm for the quantum medicine, especially in the area of aura surgery, as a logical consequence of 20 years of continuous search of side effect free, pain free, lower-cost and efficient healing methods.

www.ingramcontent.com/pod-product-compliance
Lightning Source LLC
Chambersburg PA
CBHW051732170526
45167CB00002B/902